Exercise Made Easy Guide for Seniors

Balancing Different Types of Exercises for Seniors

By

Cecil Bastien

Table of Contents

CHAPTER 1

Introduction

Welcome to the "Exercise Made Easy Guide for Seniors." This comprehensive guide is designed to empower seniors like you to embark on a journey towards a healthier and more active lifestyle through exercise. As you enter this phase of life, it's important to recognize that age is not a barrier to staying fit and enjoying the many benefits of regular physical activity. This guide will provide you with the knowledge, tips, and motivation you need to make exercise a seamless and enjoyable part of your daily routine.

1.1 Purpose of the Guide

The primary purpose of this guide is to offer seniors a reliable resource that addresses the unique considerations and challenges that come with incorporating exercise into their lives. We understand that getting started with exercise can be intimidating, especially if you're not sure where to begin or if you have concerns about your health and safety. This guide aims to demystify the process, provide clear and practical advice, and inspire confidence in your ability to take control of your physical well-being.

Throughout the pages of this guide, you'll find step-by-step instructions, expert insights, and actionable tips that cater specifically to the needs of seniors. Whether you're completely new to exercise or looking to refine your existing routine, this guide will serve as your companion, offering guidance on exercise selection, technique, safety precautions, and more. Our goal is to empower you to make informed decisions about your health and help you embrace a more active lifestyle at your own pace.

1.2 Benefits of Exercise for Seniors

Engaging in regular exercise has an array of benefits that are particularly significant for seniors. As you age, maintaining an active lifestyle becomes even more crucial for your overall well-being. Here are some of the key benefits of exercise that this guide will explore in detail:

1. **Improved Physical Health:**
   Exercise helps to maintain and
   enhance physical function. It
   strengthens muscles, bones, and
   joints, which can reduce the risk of
   falls and fractures. Additionally,
   regular exercise supports
   cardiovascular health by
   improving circulation, lowering
   blood pressure, and reducing the
   risk of chronic diseases such as
   heart disease and diabetes.

2. **Enhanced Mental Well-being:**
   Physical activity is closely linked
   to mental health. Regular exercise
   has been shown to alleviate
   symptoms of anxiety and
   depression, boost mood, and
   improve cognitive function. It
   provides a natural release of
   endorphins, often referred to as
   "feel-good" hormones, which

contribute to a positive outlook on life.

3. **Weight Management:** As metabolism tends to slow down with age, maintaining a healthy weight becomes a challenge. Exercise helps you manage your weight by burning calories, increasing muscle mass, and supporting a healthy metabolism. Combined with a balanced diet, exercise can play a crucial role in weight management.

4. **Increased Mobility and Flexibility:** Staying active helps to preserve and improve your range of motion and flexibility. This is particularly important for seniors, as it enables you to carry out daily activities with greater ease and reduces the risk of joint stiffness and muscle imbalances.

5. **Social Engagement:** Participating in group exercises, fitness classes, or recreational activities can provide opportunities for social interaction and combat feelings of isolation. Building connections and friendships through exercise can contribute to a more fulfilling and enjoyable lifestyle.

6. **Better Sleep:** Regular physical activity can positively impact your sleep patterns. Engaging in exercise promotes deeper and more restful sleep, which is essential for overall health and vitality.

7. **Enhanced Longevity:** Studies consistently show that seniors who engage in regular physical activity tend to live longer and enjoy a higher quality of life. Exercise contributes to maintaining

independence and a higher level of functional ability as you age.

This guide will delve into each of these benefits, offering insights into how exercise specifically addresses the needs and concerns of seniors. By understanding the numerous advantages of staying active, you'll be better equipped to make exercise an integral part of your daily routine.

CHAPTER 2

Getting Started

Embarking on a journey toward a more active lifestyle is an exciting endeavor, and the "Getting Started" section of this guide will serve as your compass in navigating the initial steps of your fitness journey. Whether you're completely new to exercise or returning after a hiatus, these fundamental considerations will set the stage for a successful and fulfilling experience.

2.1 Consulting Your Healthcare Provider

Before engaging in any new exercise regimen, it's crucial to consult your healthcare provider. While exercise is generally beneficial for seniors, individual health conditions and medical histories can influence the types and intensity of exercises that are safe for you. Your healthcare provider can offer personalized recommendations based on your current health status, medications, and any existing medical conditions.

During your consultation, communicate your intentions to become more physically active. Your healthcare provider can help identify any potential limitations or precautions to take into account. They can also provide insights into exercises that align with your health goals and make recommendations for adaptations if needed. This step ensures that you embark on a fitness program that is safe and tailored to your unique needs, minimizing the risk of injury or exacerbating any existing conditions.

2.2 Setting Realistic Goals

As you begin your fitness journey, setting realistic and achievable goals is essential for maintaining motivation and tracking your progress. Your goals should be specific, measurable, attainable, relevant, and time-bound (SMART). Whether your objectives are centered around weight loss, increased flexibility, improved cardiovascular health, or simply feeling more energized, having well-defined goals will help you stay focused and celebrate your successes along the way.

It's important to set both short-term and long-term goals. Short-term goals could involve establishing a consistent exercise routine, while long-term goals might encompass milestones such as completing a certain number of steps in a week or comfortably participating in a fitness class. Remember that progress is not always linear, and it's okay to adjust your goals as you gain experience and insight into what works best for you.

2.3 Importance of Warm-up and Cool-down

Before diving into your workout, it's crucial to understand the significance of warming up and cooling down. These pre- and post-exercise routines are often overlooked but play a vital role in preventing injury and optimizing the benefits of your workout.

Warm-up: A proper warm-up gradually elevates your heart rate, increases blood flow to your muscles, and prepares your body for more intense activity. Gentle cardiovascular exercises, such as brisk walking or cycling, along with dynamic stretches, can effectively warm up your muscles and joints. Warming up helps reduce the risk of strains, sprains, and other injuries that might occur if you suddenly engage in vigorous exercise without preparing your body.

Cool-down: After your workout, take time to cool down. This involves gradually decreasing the intensity of your exercise and incorporating static stretches. Cooling down helps prevent lightheadedness, gradually lowers your heart rate, and aids in the removal of waste products from your muscles. Stretching during the cool-down phase can improve flexibility and prevent post-exercise muscle tightness.

Incorporating warm-up and cool-down routines into your exercise sessions, you create a foundation for safe and effective workouts. These practices not only enhance your overall exercise experience but also contribute to your body's ability to recover and adapt to the demands of physical activity.

CHAPTER 3

Types of Exercises for Seniors

3.1 Aerobic/Cardiovascular Exercises

Aerobic or cardiovascular exercises are activities that get your heart pumping, improve circulation, and boost your overall cardiovascular fitness. Engaging in regular aerobic exercises can lead to increased endurance, improved lung capacity, and a healthier heart.

3.1.1 Walking

Walking is a low-impact exercise that is accessible to almost everyone. It requires minimal equipment and can be done indoors on a treadmill or outdoors in your neighborhood or local park. Aim for brisk walking to elevate your heart rate and engage your muscles. Walking is not only great for cardiovascular health but also provides an opportunity for social interaction and exposure to nature.

3.1.2 Swimming

Swimming is a fantastic full-body workout that is easy on the joints. The buoyancy of water reduces the impact on your muscles and bones, making it an ideal option for seniors with joint issues or mobility challenges. Swimming improves cardiovascular fitness, strengthens muscles, and enhances flexibility.

3.1.3 Cycling

Cycling, whether on a stationary bike or outdoors, is an excellent way to improve cardiovascular health and lower body strength. It's a low-impact exercise that allows you to control the intensity of your workout. Cycling also provides an opportunity to explore your surroundings and enjoy the outdoors.

3.2 Strength Training

Strength training is essential for maintaining muscle mass, bone density, and overall functional capacity as you age. It can improve your ability to perform daily activities and enhance your metabolism.

3.2.1 Bodyweight Exercises

Bodyweight exercises use your own body weight as resistance to build strength. Examples include squats, lunges, push-ups, and planks. These exercises can be modified to suit your fitness level and can be performed at home or in a gym.

3.2.2 Resistance Bands

Resistance bands are versatile tools that provide resistance throughout the full range of motion. They are gentle on the joints and can be used to target various muscle groups. Resistance bands come in different levels of resistance, allowing you to gradually increase the intensity of your workouts.

3.2.3 Light Weights

Using light weights or dumbbells is another effective way to engage in strength training. Start with a weight that feels comfortable and gradually increase it as you become stronger. Focus on proper form and controlled movements to prevent injury.

Incorporating a combination of aerobic and strength training exercises into your routine can provide a well-rounded approach to fitness. Remember that it's important to start at a level that is appropriate for your current fitness level and gradually progress as you become more comfortable and confident.

3.3 Flexibility and Balance Exercises

Flexibility and balance are crucial components of functional fitness, especially as we age. Incorporating flexibility and balance exercises into your routine can help improve your posture, prevent injuries, and enhance your overall mobility.

3.3.1 Stretching

Stretching exercises are designed to increase the flexibility of your muscles and joints. Regular stretching can help alleviate muscle tension, improve your range of motion, and reduce the risk of strains and injuries. Here are a few types of stretching exercises to consider:

- **Static Stretching:** Hold a stretch in a comfortable position for 15-30 seconds without bouncing. Focus on major muscle groups like hamstrings, quadriceps, calves, and shoulders.

- **Dynamic Stretching:** Incorporate gentle movements to warm up your muscles before static stretching. Examples include arm swings, leg swings, and hip circles.

- **Proprioceptive Neuromuscular Facilitation (PNF):** This involves a combination of stretching and contracting muscles. It's often done with a partner, but self-assisted PNF stretches can also be effective.

3.3.2 Yoga

Yoga is a holistic practice that combines physical postures, breathing exercises, and meditation. It enhances flexibility, balance, and strength while promoting relaxation and stress reduction. Many yoga classes cater specifically to seniors, focusing on gentle poses and modifications to accommodate different abilities.

- **Hatha Yoga:** A gentle and slower-paced form of yoga that emphasizes basic poses, alignment, and breath control.

- **Chair Yoga:** This variation of yoga is done while seated or using a chair for support. It's ideal for seniors with limited mobility or balance concerns.

- **Restorative Yoga:** Involves holding poses for longer periods, using props for support. It's deeply relaxing and can be especially beneficial for reducing stress.

3.3.3 Tai Chi

Tai Chi is a mind-body practice that originated as a martial art in China. It consists of slow, flowing movements that promote balance, flexibility, and relaxation. Tai Chi is particularly beneficial for improving coordination and reducing the risk of falls. It can be adapted to different fitness levels and is often practiced in groups.

The combination of stretching, yoga, and Tai Chi provides a comprehensive approach to enhancing flexibility and balance. These exercises not only contribute to physical well-being but also support mental clarity and a sense of calm. As you incorporate flexibility and balance exercises into your routine, you'll notice improvements in your overall mobility and a greater sense of control over your body.

CHAPTER 4

Designing Your Exercise Routine

Creating a well-structured exercise routine is essential for making consistent progress, preventing burnout, and enjoying a balanced fitness journey.

4.1 Creating a Weekly Schedule

Establishing a weekly exercise schedule helps you stay organized and committed to your fitness goals. Consider the following steps when designing your weekly exercise plan:

1. **Assess Your Availability:**
   Determine how many days per
   week you can realistically dedicate
   to exercise. Keep in mind that
   consistency is more important than
   the number of days.

2. **Plan for Variety:** Aim for a mix
   of aerobic, strength, flexibility, and
   balance exercises. This variety
   ensures that you address different
   aspects of fitness and prevent
   overuse injuries.

3. **Gradual Progression:** If you're
   new to exercise, start with 2-3 days
   per week and gradually increase
   the frequency. Allow your body
   time to adapt and recover.

4. **Rest and Recovery:** Include rest
   days to allow your muscles to
   recover. These days are crucial for
   preventing fatigue and injury.

5. **Duration and Intensity:**
   Gradually increase the duration
   and intensity of your workouts
   over time. Listen to your body and
   avoid pushing yourself too hard.

6. **Social and Fun Activities:**
   Incorporate activities you enjoy
   and can do with friends or family.
   This boosts motivation and adds a
   social element to your routine.

7. **Flexibility:** Be open to adjusting
   your schedule as needed. Life can
   be unpredictable, so having a
   flexible approach is important.

4.2 Balancing Different Types of Exercises

Balancing different types of exercises
is key to achieving a well-rounded
fitness routine that addresses various

aspects of your health. Consider the following categories when structuring your routine:

1. **Aerobic/Cardiovascular Exercises:** Include 2-3 sessions of moderate-intensity aerobic exercise per week. This could involve activities like brisk walking, swimming, or cycling.

2. **Strength Training:** Aim for 2-3 strength training sessions per week, targeting major muscle groups. Alternating between different exercises can prevent overuse injuries and keep your routine engaging.

3. **Flexibility and Balance:** Incorporate stretching, yoga, or Tai Chi into your routine 2-3 times per week. These exercises improve

your flexibility, balance, and overall mobility.

4. **Rest and Active Recovery:** Allow for at least 1-2 days of rest or active recovery, such as light walking or gentle stretching. Rest is essential for muscle repair and preventing burnout.

5. **Progression:** Gradually increase the intensity, duration, and complexity of your workouts as your fitness level improves. This progression keeps your body challenged and ensures continued growth.

6. **Listen to Your Body:** Pay attention to how your body responds to different exercises. If you experience pain or discomfort, modify the exercise or seek professional guidance.

The best exercise routine is one that you can stick to and enjoy. Be patient with yourself, and don't hesitate to make adjustments as you discover what works best for you.

4.3 Progression and Adaptation

As you engage in regular exercise, the concept of progression and adaptation becomes central to your journey. Progression involves gradually increasing the intensity, duration, or complexity of your workouts over time, while adaptation refers to your body's response to the physical demands placed upon it. By understanding these concepts, you can optimize your fitness gains and continue to challenge yourself in a safe and effective manner.

Progression Strategies:

1. **Gradual Intensity Increase:**
   When you're comfortable with a
   certain exercise, gradually increase
   the intensity. For example, if
   you're walking, try picking up the
   pace or adding short intervals of
   brisk walking.

2. **Incremental Reps and Sets:** In
   strength training, aim to gradually
   increase the number of repetitions
   (reps) or sets you perform for each
   exercise. This helps build muscular
   strength and endurance.

3. **Resistance Increment:** If using
   resistance bands or weights,
   gradually increase the resistance as
   your strength improves. This
   ensures ongoing muscle
   development.

4. **Extended Workout Duration:** As your cardiovascular fitness improves, extend the duration of your aerobic exercises. Add a few extra minutes to your walks, swims, or cycling sessions.

5. **Advanced Exercises:** Once you've mastered basic exercises, consider progressing to more advanced variations that challenge your muscles and coordination.

Adaptation and Recovery:

1. **Rest and Recovery:** Your body needs time to recover and adapt to the stress of exercise. Adequate sleep, proper nutrition, and rest days are essential for optimal adaptation.

2. **Muscle Soreness:** Mild muscle soreness after a workout is normal, but severe or prolonged pain could

indicate overexertion or improper form. Listen to your body and adjust accordingly.

3. **Plateaus:** It's common to experience plateaus in your progress. If you find that you're no longer seeing improvements, it might be time to adjust your routine or add new exercises.

4. **Incorporate Variety:** To continue challenging your body and preventing boredom, incorporate different exercises, change up your routine, or explore new fitness activities.

5. **Listen to Your Body:** If you experience pain, fatigue, or other unusual symptoms, it's important to listen to your body and consult a healthcare professional if necessary.

Staying Mindful:

1. **Keep a Workout Journal:**
   Record your exercises, sets, reps, and any notes about how you felt during the workout. This can help you track your progress and make informed adjustments.

2. **Body Awareness:** Pay attention to how your body responds to exercise. Be mindful of any discomfort, fatigue, or changes in energy levels.

3. **Celebrate Achievements:**
   Celebrate your achievements, no matter how small. Progress is a journey, and acknowledging your successes keeps you motivated.

4. **Reassess Goals:** Periodically reassess your fitness goals and adjust your routine accordingly. This prevents complacency and

keeps you focused on continuous improvement.

Incorporating progressive strategies and staying adaptable to the changing needs of your body, you can ensure that your exercise routine remains effective and enjoyable.

CHAPTER 5

Exercise Safety Tips

Prioritizing safety during your exercise routine is paramount to preventing injuries and enjoying a sustainable fitness journey. By following these safety tips, you can create a secure and effective workout environment that supports your overall well-being.

5.1 Proper Form and Technique

Maintaining proper form and technique during exercises is crucial for preventing injuries and maximizing the effectiveness of your workouts. Here's how to ensure proper form:

1. **Start Slowly:** Begin with lighter weights or lower resistance to focus on form before increasing intensity.

2. **Focus on Alignment:** Pay attention to your body's alignment during exercises. Keep your spine neutral, shoulders relaxed, and engage your core muscles.

3. **Use Controlled Movements:** Avoid jerky or sudden movements. Perform exercises with controlled and deliberate motions.

4. **Breathe:** Breathe naturally throughout the exercise. Exhale during the exertion phase and inhale during the relaxation phase.

5. **Consult Professionals:** If you're unsure about proper form, consider working with a fitness trainer or instructor who can provide guidance.

5.2 Using Appropriate Equipment

Using the right equipment and ensuring its proper setup is essential for a safe workout experience:

1. **Choose the Right Shoes:** Wear supportive and properly fitting shoes that match the activity. Proper footwear helps prevent strains and provides stability.

2. **Check Equipment Safety:** Ensure that exercise equipment is in good condition and properly maintained.

Check for any loose parts or wear and tear.

3. **Use Safety Features:** When using gym equipment, familiarize yourself with safety features and proper usage instructions.

4. **Gradually Introduce New Equipment:** If incorporating new equipment, start with lower resistance or weights to acquaint yourself with proper usage and prevent accidents.

5.3 Listening to Your Body

Listening to your body and respecting its signals is essential for staying safe during exercise:

1. **Warm-Up and Cool-Down:**
Prioritize warm-up exercises
before your main workout and
cool-down stretches afterward.

2. **Pay Attention to Pain:**
Distinguish between discomfort
(normal during exercise) and pain
(indicative of injury). Stop any
exercise that causes pain.

3. **Rest and Recovery:** Allow
adequate time for rest and recovery
between workouts. Overtraining
can lead to injuries and burnout.

4. **Stay Hydrated:** Drink water
before, during, and after your
workout to stay hydrated.

5. **Modify as Needed:** If an exercise
feels too challenging or
uncomfortable, modify it to match
your fitness level.

6. **Consult a Professional:** If you
    have health concerns or are new to
    exercise, consult your healthcare
    provider before starting a new
    routine.

Practicing proper form, using
appropriate equipment, and tuning in
to your body's cues, you can
significantly reduce the risk of
injuries and ensure a safe and
enjoyable exercise experience.

CHAPTER 6

Staying Motivated

Maintaining motivation is a crucial factor in sustaining an active and healthy lifestyle. While there may be days when your enthusiasm wanes, implementing strategies to keep yourself engaged and excited about exercise can help you overcome challenges and stay on track.

6.1 Finding Enjoyable Activities

Discovering exercises and activities that you genuinely enjoy can make a significant difference in your motivation to stay active:

1. **Try New Things:** Experiment with various types of exercises until you find ones that resonate with you. Whether it's dancing, hiking, or playing a sport, finding something you love makes it easier to commit.

2. **Set Goals:** Set specific goals that align with your interests. For instance, if you enjoy walking, you might aim to complete a certain number of steps or explore new walking routes.

3. **Variety:** Mix up your routine to prevent boredom. Incorporate different exercises, environments, and workout formats to keep things fresh.

4. **Outdoor Activities:** Nature offers a beautiful backdrop for exercise. Try outdoor activities like hiking,

gardening, or even practicing yoga in a park.

5. **Reward Yourself:** Celebrate your achievements with rewards that don't undermine your progress. Treat yourself to a favorite book, a movie night, or a relaxing bath.

6.2 Exercising with Friends and Family

Exercising with others can make your fitness journey more enjoyable and provide built-in accountability:

1. **Social Support:** Partnering with friends or family members can make workouts more enjoyable. You can motivate each other, share tips, and celebrate successes together.

2. **Group Activities:** Join group fitness classes, walking clubs, or sports leagues. Participating in group activities fosters a sense of community and camaraderie.

3. **Workout Buddies:** Having a workout buddy helps you stay committed. You're less likely to skip a workout if you know someone is counting on you.

4. **Friendly Competition:** Friendly competition can be a fun way to push yourself. Set challenges or goals with your exercise companions.

5. **Quality Time:** Exercising with loved ones allows you to spend quality time together while prioritizing your health.

Motivation can ebb and flow, so it's important to be patient with yourself.

By incorporating enjoyable activities and involving friends or family in your fitness routine, you create an environment that fosters long-term commitment and enthusiasm.

6.3 Tracking Your Progress

Tracking your progress is a valuable tool for staying motivated and monitoring the results of your efforts. Whether you're aiming to improve your strength, endurance, flexibility, or overall well-being, keeping track of your achievements can provide a sense of accomplishment and help you make informed decisions about your fitness journey.

Why Track Your Progress:

1. **Visual Feedback:** Progress tracking provides a visual record of your improvements over time. Seeing tangible results can be incredibly motivating.

2. **Goal Assessment:** Regularly assessing your progress helps you determine whether you're on track to meet your goals or if adjustments are needed.

3. **Boosted Motivation:** Celebrating small victories boosts your motivation to continue exercising and maintain a healthy lifestyle.

4. **Identify Trends:** Tracking can help you identify patterns, such as which exercises or routines yield the best results for you.

5. **Accountability:** Monitoring your progress adds a level of accountability, as you're more

likely to stick to your routine when you have a clear record of your efforts.

How to Track Your Progress:

1. **Keep a Workout Journal:** Record each workout, including exercises performed, sets, reps, and any notes about how you felt during the session.

2. **Take Measurements:** Track measurements like weight, body measurements (waist, hips, etc.), and body composition changes over time.

3. **Use Fitness Apps:** Numerous fitness apps allow you to log workouts, track progress, and set reminders for your exercise sessions.

4. **Photographic Evidence:** Take regular photos to visually document your progress. Compare photos from different time periods to see visible changes.

5. **Track Performance:** If you're focused on strength or endurance improvements, track metrics such as the weight lifted, the number of repetitions, or the time taken to complete a certain distance.

6. **Set Milestones:** Set specific milestones and celebrate reaching them. For instance, if you're working on flexibility, celebrate when you can touch your toes comfortably.

7. **Listen to Your Body:** While tracking is important, also listen to your body. If you're feeling

fatigued, give yourself permission to take a step back.

Review and Adjust:

Regularly review your progress to identify trends, areas of improvement, and achievements. If you notice a plateau or want to accelerate your progress, consider adjusting your routine, increasing intensity, or trying new exercises.

progress is a personal journey, and there's no one-size-fits-all approach. Embrace the uniqueness of your fitness journey and take pride in the steps you've taken toward a healthier lifestyle.

CHAPTER 7

Incorporating Exercise into Daily Life

Making exercise a habit is essential for long-term success. When exercise becomes a consistent part of your daily routine, it becomes easier to stay motivated and enjoy the many benefits of an active lifestyle.

7.1 Making Physical Activity a Habit

Creating a habit involves consistent repetition until an action becomes automatic. Here's how to make exercise a habitual part of your daily life:

Start Small: Begin with achievable goals that require minimal time and effort. This reduces the chance of feeling overwhelmed and increases your likelihood of success.

Set a Specific Schedule: Dedicate specific times for exercise each day. Treat these times as appointments that you prioritize and stick to.

Pair with Existing Habits: Attach your exercise routine to an existing habit. For example, go for a walk after your morning coffee or do stretches while watching your favorite TV show.

Make It Enjoyable: Choose activities you genuinely enjoy. If you look forward to your workout, you're more likely to stick with it.

Create Reminders: Set alarms, reminders, or calendar events to prompt you to exercise. This helps establish a routine until it becomes second nature.

Track Your Progress: Monitoring your consistency helps reinforce your commitment. Use a workout journal or an app to log your sessions.

Reward Yourself: Celebrate your milestones with small rewards. It could be treating yourself to a favorite healthy snack or enjoying a relaxing evening after a productive workout.

Stay Flexible: While routine is important, life can be unpredictable. If you miss a scheduled workout, don't get discouraged; simply resume your routine the next day.

Practice Self-Compassion: Be kind to yourself on days when motivation is low. If you miss a session, avoid self-criticism and remember that tomorrow is a new opportunity.

Social Accountability: Share your goals with friends or family who can provide support and encouragement. You can even consider an exercise buddy to keep you accountable.

Visualize Success: Imagine the positive outcomes of consistent exercise—increased energy, improved health, and a sense of accomplishment.

Forming a habit takes time. Be patient with yourself and recognize that small, consistent efforts lead to significant results. By integrating exercise into your daily routine, you're fostering a healthier and more active lifestyle that benefits your overall well-being.

7.2 Finding Opportunities for Movement

Incorporating movement into your daily life goes beyond structured workouts. Finding opportunities for physical activity throughout the day can contribute significantly to your overall fitness and well-being. Here are some strategies to help you stay active beyond your formal exercise routine:

Active Commuting: If possible, walk or bike to nearby destinations instead of driving. If you use public transportation, consider getting off a stop early and walking the rest of the way.

Take the Stairs: Opt for stairs instead of elevators whenever possible. Climbing stairs is a great way to engage your leg muscles and get your heart rate up.

Break Time Movement: During breaks, take a short walk, do stretches, or perform light exercises to refresh your body and mind.

Household Chores: Engage in activities like gardening, cleaning, or rearranging furniture. These tasks can provide a decent workout while accomplishing necessary chores.

Active Leisure: Choose leisure activities that involve movement, such as dancing, playing an active game with family, or going for a leisurely bike ride.

Walk and Talk: If you have phone calls to make, use the opportunity to walk while talking. This adds extra steps to your day.

Park Farther Away: When running errands, intentionally park your car farther away from the entrance to increase your walking distance.

Desk Exercises: If you have a sedentary job, incorporate desk exercises like seated leg lifts or shoulder stretches to keep your body active.

Standing Breaks: If you work at a desk, set a timer to remind you to stand up, stretch, and move around every hour.

Engage in Hobbies: Pursue hobbies that involve physical activity, whether it's dancing, gardening, or playing a musical instrument.

Family Activities: Involve your family in physical activities like family walks, bike rides, or outdoor games.

Seeking out opportunities for movement in your daily routine, you can accumulate additional physical activity that complements your structured workouts. These small changes add up over time and contribute to improved cardiovascular health, increased energy expenditure, and enhanced overall fitness.

7.3 Combining Exercise with Daily Tasks

Efficiency is key in today's busy world, and combining exercise with daily tasks is a smart way to maximize your time and incorporate physical activity seamlessly into your routine. Here's how you can blend exercise with your everyday tasks:

Walking Meetings: If possible, schedule walking meetings instead of sitting in a conference room. Walking and talking can boost creativity and productivity.

Active Commuting: Choose to walk or bike to work if feasible. Alternatively, if you use public transportation, consider walking to a farther stop before getting on.

Kitchen Workouts: While waiting for water to boil or food to cook, do quick exercises like squats, calf raises, or leg lifts.

Stair Climbing Breaks: If you're at home or work, take mini stair-climbing breaks throughout the day. A few trips up and down the stairs can add up.

Lunchtime Walks: Use your lunch break for a brisk walk around your workplace or nearby park. This can be refreshing and improve concentration in the afternoon.

TV Time Workouts: During TV commercials, perform bodyweight exercises like push-ups, planks, or lunges.

Desk Exercise Breaks: Incorporate short exercise breaks into your workday. Do seated leg lifts, shoulder stretches, or desk push-ups.

Multitasking Squats: While brushing your teeth or waiting for something to microwave, do a few squats to engage your leg muscles.

Waiting Room Stretches: If you find yourself waiting in a queue or sitting in a waiting room, use the time to stretch your muscles.

Active Cleaning: Turn cleaning into a workout by adding lunges, squats, or twists while vacuuming, sweeping, or doing laundry.

Gardening as Exercise: Gardening involves a variety of physical movements such as bending, lifting, and digging. It's a great way to get both exercise and fresh air.

merging exercise with daily tasks, you're optimizing your time and ensuring that physical activity becomes an integral part of your routine. These small adjustments can make a significant difference in your overall fitness levels while accommodating your busy lifestyle.

CHAPTER 8

Nutrition and Hydration

Maintaining a balanced diet and staying hydrated are essential components of supporting your overall health and optimizing your exercise performance. Proper nutrition provides your body with the energy and nutrients it needs to function effectively.

8.1 Importance of a Balanced Diet

A balanced diet is one that provides your body with the right amount of nutrients from various food groups.

Here's why it's crucial for supporting your exercise and overall well-being:

Fueling Your Workouts: Carbohydrates are your body's primary source of energy. They provide the fuel needed for both aerobic and strength training exercises. Including complex carbohydrates like whole grains, fruits, and vegetables in your diet ensures sustained energy levels.

Muscle Repair and Growth: Protein is essential for muscle repair and growth, especially after strength training workouts. Incorporate lean sources of protein like poultry, fish, beans, and legumes into your meals.

Recovery and Immunity: Vitamins and minerals are vital for recovery and maintaining a strong immune system. Colorful fruits and vegetables are rich in antioxidants, which help combat oxidative stress caused by exercise.

Bone Health: Adequate calcium and vitamin D intake supports bone health, which is particularly important for seniors. Dairy products, leafy greens, and fortified foods are good sources.

Hydration: Staying hydrated is essential for optimal exercise performance. Water helps regulate body temperature, transport nutrients, and remove waste products. Drink water before, during, and after exercise.

Balanced Meals: Aim for balanced meals that include a combination of carbohydrates, protein, and healthy fats. This balance provides sustained energy, stabilizes blood sugar levels, and supports satiety.

Eating Before Exercise: Have a light, balanced meal or snack before exercising, especially if your workout is scheduled a couple of hours after a meal. This provides energy without causing discomfort.

Eating After Exercise: Consume a meal or snack containing both protein and carbohydrates within the first hour after exercise. This aids in muscle recovery and replenishes glycogen stores.

Individual Needs: Nutrition is highly individual. Consult a registered dietitian or healthcare provider for personalized dietary recommendations based on your goals, activity level, and any specific health conditions.

No single food or supplement can replace the benefits of a balanced diet. A diverse range of nutrient-rich foods provides your body with the necessary building blocks for overall health, exercise performance, and well-being.

8.2 Pre- and Post-Exercise Nutrition

Proper nutrition before and after exercise plays a significant role in maximizing your workout performance, promoting recovery, and supporting your overall health. Understanding what to eat and when can help you get the most out of your exercise routine.

Pre-Exercise Nutrition:

Eating the right foods before a workout provides your body with the necessary energy and nutrients to perform at its best. Consider these guidelines for pre-exercise nutrition:

Timing: Aim to eat a balanced meal or snack about 1-2 hours before your workout. This gives your body enough time to digest the food and convert it into usable energy.

Carbohydrates: Choose complex carbohydrates such as whole grains, fruits, and vegetables. These provide a steady release of energy during your workout.

Protein: Include a small amount of protein to support muscle repair and maintenance. Options like yogurt, lean meats, or plant-based sources like beans and lentils are good choices.

Hydration: Drink water to ensure you're well-hydrated before starting your exercise. Dehydration can negatively impact performance.

Avoid High-Fat and High-Fiber Foods: These foods can cause discomfort during exercise due to slower digestion.

Sample Pre-Exercise Snacks:

- Greek yogurt with berries and a sprinkle of granola

- Banana with a tablespoon of nut butter

- Whole grain toast with turkey and veggies

Post-Exercise Nutrition:

After your workout, providing your body with the right nutrients helps with recovery and muscle repair. Here are some tips for post-exercise nutrition:

Timing: Consume a meal or snack containing carbohydrates and protein within an hour after your workout. This window is when your muscles are most receptive to nutrient uptake.

Carbohydrates: Replenish glycogen stores by consuming carbohydrates. Opt for whole grains, fruits, and starchy vegetables.

Protein: Protein is crucial for muscle repair and growth. Include lean sources such as chicken, fish, eggs, or plant-based options like tofu.

Hydration: Rehydrate by drinking water after your workout. If it was a particularly intense session, consider beverages with added electrolytes.

Sample Post-Exercise Meals:

- Grilled chicken with quinoa and roasted vegetables

- Whole grain pasta with marinara sauce and lean ground turkey

- Smoothie with spinach, banana, protein powder, and almond milk

Remember that individual needs vary based on factors like exercise intensity, duration, and personal preferences. Experiment with different foods and timing to find what works best for you. Consulting a registered dietitian can provide personalized recommendations to support your fitness goals.

8.3 Hydration Tips for Seniors

Staying properly hydrated is essential for seniors, especially when engaging in physical activity and exercise. As we age, our body's natural thirst signals may become less effective, making it crucial to be proactive about hydration. Here are some hydration tips tailored to seniors:

1. Drink Throughout the Day: Don't rely solely on feeling thirsty. Set a schedule to drink water regularly, even if you don't feel thirsty.

2. Monitor Urine Color: Use urine color as a general indicator of hydration. Pale yellow to light straw is a sign of good hydration, while dark yellow or amber can indicate dehydration.

3. Stay Hydrated Before Exercise: Drink water before you start your workout to ensure you're properly hydrated. Dehydration can affect exercise performance and increase the risk of injury.

4. Sip During Exercise: Bring a water bottle and take sips during your exercise session, especially if it's hot or humid. Aim to drink every 15-20 minutes.

5. Choose Water-Rich Foods: Incorporate foods with high water content, such as fruits (watermelon, oranges, and grapes) and vegetables (cucumbers, lettuce, and celery).

6. Avoid Excessive Caffeine and Alcohol: Both caffeine and alcohol can contribute to dehydration. If you consume these beverages, balance them with water intake.

7. Set Reminders: Use alarms, apps, or sticky notes as reminders to drink water regularly throughout the day.

8. Use a Reusable Water Bottle: Having a water bottle with you makes it easier to track your water intake and stay hydrated on the go.

9. Hydration with Meals: Drink water before, during, and after meals to support digestion and overall hydration.

10. Be Mindful of Medications: Some medications can impact your body's fluid balance. Consult your healthcare provider to understand how your medications may affect hydration.

11. Listen to Your Body: Pay attention to signs of dehydration, such as dry mouth, dark urine, dizziness, and fatigue. Address these symptoms promptly.

12. Hydration for Exercise Recovery: After exercising, rehydrate with water and consider beverages with added electrolytes if you've had a particularly intense workout.

13. Consider Electrolyte Intake: Include foods with natural electrolytes, such as potassium-rich bananas or sodium-containing broth, to help maintain electrolyte balance.

Staying hydrated is an important aspect of maintaining overall health and well-being, especially as a senior. By being proactive about your fluid intake and incorporating these hydration tips into your routine, you can ensure that your body is properly nourished and ready to take on physical activities and exercise.

CHAPTER 9

Overcoming Barriers

As you pursue an active and healthy lifestyle, you may encounter various barriers that can hinder your progress. It's important to recognize these challenges and find strategies to overcome them.

9.1 Addressing Time Constraints

Busy schedules and time constraints are common challenges that many individuals face when trying to incorporate exercise into their lives. Here's how to overcome this barrier:

Prioritize: Make exercise a priority by scheduling it into your day just like you would any other important task. Consider it non-negotiable.

Break It Up: If you can't find a continuous block of time for exercise, break it up into shorter sessions throughout the day. Even 10-minute bouts of activity add up.

Combine Tasks: Find ways to combine exercise with daily tasks. For example, you can do bodyweight exercises while watching TV or take a brisk walk during your lunch break.

Early Mornings: Consider waking up a bit earlier to fit in your workout before the day gets busy. Morning exercise can set a positive tone for the rest of the day.

Lunchtime Workouts: Use your lunch break for a quick workout. This can help you recharge and boost your energy for the afternoon.

Involve Others: Engage family members or friends in your workouts. Exercising together can make it a fun and social activity.

Maximize Efficiency: Choose workouts that provide the most benefit in a shorter amount of time. High-intensity interval training (HIIT) is a great option for time-efficient workouts.

Plan Ahead: Set aside time at the beginning of the week to plan your workouts. Having a clear plan makes it easier to follow through.

Be Realistic: You don't need hours of exercise each day. Aim for at least 150 minutes of moderate-intensity aerobic activity per week, and break it down as needed.

Embrace Flexibility: If your schedule gets disrupted, don't stress. Adjust your routine and make the most of the time you have.

consistency is key. Even small amounts of regular physical activity can contribute to improved health and fitness. By finding creative ways to fit exercise into your busy schedule, you're taking a proactive step toward prioritizing your well-being.

9.2 Dealing with Limited Mobility

Limited mobility can present unique challenges, but it doesn't have to be a barrier to staying active. There are plenty of exercises and activities that can be adapted to accommodate different levels of mobility. Here's how to navigate this challenge:

Consult a Professional: Before starting any new exercise routine, especially if you have mobility limitations, consult with your healthcare provider or a physical therapist. They can provide guidance tailored to your specific needs and abilities.

Seated Exercises: Many exercises can be performed while seated, making them accessible for individuals with limited mobility.

Seated leg lifts, seated marches, and seated twists are examples of exercises that engage various muscle groups.

Resistance Bands: Resistance bands are versatile and can provide resistance for strength training exercises even when seated. They're gentle on joints and can help improve muscle strength.

Chair Yoga: Chair yoga focuses on gentle stretches and poses that can be done while sitting in a chair. It improves flexibility, balance, and relaxation.

Aquatic Exercise: If possible, consider water-based activities. Water buoyancy reduces impact on joints and provides resistance for strengthening exercises.

Balance Exercises: Even if mobility is limited, working on balance is important. Standing on one leg (with support if needed), leg lifts, and toe taps can help improve balance.

Range of Motion Exercises: Incorporate exercises that focus on improving joint mobility. Arm circles, ankle pumps, and wrist stretches can help maintain flexibility.

Modify Intensity: Tailor exercises to your comfort level. If an exercise feels too challenging, modify it or reduce the intensity. Always prioritize safety and avoid pain.

Mindful Movement: Engage in activities like tai chi or gentle stretching that focus on mindful movement and promote relaxation.

Utilize Supportive Aids: If needed, use assistive devices such as canes, walkers, or support bars to ensure safety while exercising.

Set Realistic Goals: Focus on what you can do and set achievable goals that align with your current abilities.

Stay Positive: Embrace the progress you make and celebrate small victories along the way.

Every person's journey is unique. The key is to find exercises and activities that work for you and support your mobility needs. With the right guidance and adaptations, you can maintain an active lifestyle and continue to experience the benefits of regular physical activity.

9.3 Handling Weather and Environmental Factors

Weather and environmental conditions can sometimes pose challenges to staying active. However, with a bit of flexibility and planning, you can continue to engage in physical activity regardless of the conditions. Here's how to navigate weather and environmental factors:

Hot Weather:

- **Stay Hydrated:** Drink water before, during, and after your workout, especially in hot weather.

- **Time It Right:** Exercise during cooler parts of the day, such as early morning or late evening.

- **Wear Lightweight Clothing:** Opt for moisture-wicking fabrics that keep you cool and comfortable.

- **Protect Your Skin:** Wear sunscreen, a hat, and sunglasses to shield yourself from the sun.

- **Choose Indoor Activities:** If it's too hot outside, consider indoor activities like dancing, swimming, or using a treadmill.

Cold Weather:

- **Layer Up:** Wear layers of clothing to trap warmth and adjust as needed.

- **Warm-Up Thoroughly:** Spend extra time warming up your muscles to prevent injury in cold temperatures.

- **Stay Visible:** If exercising outdoors in low light, wear reflective clothing or accessories for visibility.

- **Keep Hydrated:** Even in cold weather, staying hydrated is essential.

- **Be Cautious of Icy Conditions:** If it's icy or slippery, opt for indoor exercises to avoid falls.

Rainy Weather:

- **Stay Dry:** Wear waterproof clothing to stay dry during your workout.

- **Choose Indoor Workouts:** If the weather is stormy, consider indoor exercises or activities.

- **Be Cautious of Slippery Surfaces:** Rain can create

slippery surfaces, so choose paths or areas that are less affected by puddles.

Environmental Concerns:

- **Air Quality:** On days with poor air quality, opt for indoor workouts to minimize exposure to pollutants.

- **Allergies:** If you have allergies, check pollen counts and choose activities that reduce exposure to allergens.

- **Wildlife and Insects:** In certain areas, wildlife or insects can be a concern. Plan your activities accordingly.

Adapt and Adjust:

Remember that flexibility is key. If weather conditions make outdoor exercise challenging, explore indoor options like home workouts, gym sessions, or fitness classes. If you're determined to exercise outdoors, be prepared with appropriate clothing and gear.

Safety First:

Prioritize safety above all else. If weather conditions pose a risk to your safety or health, it's best to stay indoors or find alternative activities.

Being adaptable and proactive, you can continue your fitness routine regardless of the weather or environmental factors. Staying active in different conditions not only supports your physical health but also showcases your commitment to your well-being.